THE SPANISH FLU IN RETROSPECT:

A Brief History and LESSONS FROM THE TWENTIETH CENTURY PANDEMIC |
Great Influenza 1918

James Walter

ISBN: 978-1-950284-98-6

ISBN: 978-1-950284-98-6

Table of Contents

Table of Contents...3

OTHER INTRESTING READS...........................4

INTRODUCTION 5

Chapter 1: The Brief History of the Spanish Flu...........8

    What Is the Spanish Flu?...........................8

    The emergence of the Flu 9

    Why Called Spanish...................................11

    Spanish Flu Symptoms 12

Chapter 2: The Deadliest Plague in History...............14

Chapter 3: The Spanish Flu and the Years After 22

    An Unforgettable Failure of Medical Scientists 22

    Fighting the Flu 23

    Aspirin Came Promising but Poisoning 24

    Spanish Flu Pandemic Ends.........................26

Chapter 4: Lessons From the Spanish Flu Outbreak ...27

    Some of the Lessons for Our Day.................27

    Another Pandemic Coming? 30

    Avoiding the Next Pandemic........................32

CONCLUSIONS..33

OTHER INTRESTING READS

Are you worried about the present virus pandemic and wish to arm yourself with enough information from the past? Get the books below, sit back, relax and BE INFORMED!

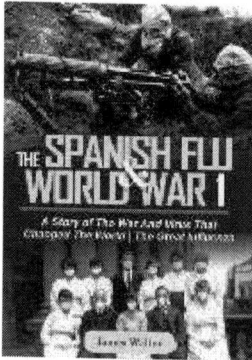

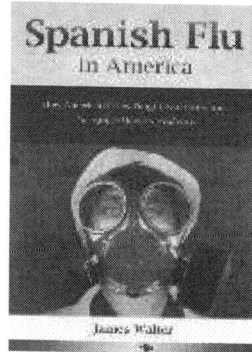

mybook.to/spanishflu2 | mybook.to/spanishflu3

INTRODUCTION

Pandemic is anything but new to human society. Scientists at different ages have been shocked, baffled, and had struggled to cope with various deadly infectious diseases throughout centuries.

The earliest pandemic in the acceptable recorded history occurred in 430 B.C. It was reported to have broken out in Athens during or after the Peloponnesian War. The disease, believed to be typhoid fever, quickly spread to African countries of Egypt, Ethiopia, and Libya. It brought along symptoms such as fever, redskin, thirst, and blood in the throat and tongue. Historians claim that the havoc it wreaked on the Athenians was a big factor contributing to their fall to the Spartans.

Since then, the world has been visited by the Antonine Plague which occurred in 165AD. It took 5 million lives across Asia, Egypt, Greece, and Italy. Less than 400 years later, around 541-542 AD, the Plague of Justinian also swept away 25 million in just 12 months.

Over 1000 years later the Black Death pandemic was reported to have started from China. 10 million Indians succumbed to the plague between 1346 and 1353. The 7-year-long pandemic was caused by bubonic plague later discovered to be transmitted by fleas. The estimated population of the world then was 400 million and Black Death reduced it by half. The 200 million people that survived it were convinced that this world could no longer be ended a disease.

Even then, the Third Cholera pandemic threatened to wipe away humans by killing over 1 million people in a scourge that lasted from 1852 to 1860. The pandemic started in India and spread from the Ganges River Delta through Asia, Europe, the Americas, and Africa

Toward the end of the 19th century, the world witnessed yet another pandemic which also claimed over 1 million lives. It was the "Asiatic Flu" or "Russian Flu" that broke out first in May 1889 in three different locations. Reports of the outbreak of the disease came simultaneously from distant Bukhara in Central Asia (now Turkestan), Canada, and Greenland. It didn't take long before it spread worldwide. It taught the world a lot about bacteriology.

Let's now shift the attention to a more recent pandemic that marred the 20th century at the onset. We are not talking about HIV/AIDs here. We are looking at what is known as the Spanish flu. This is another dreadful pandemic that will not be forgotten in haste.

What is the Spanish flu? When did it break out? What caused the outbreak? Where did it start? What was the fatality figure? How was it contained? Is there anything significant about this flu that's still relevant for our day? If there is, what lessons can be taken away from its history?

This book has been entirely devoted to the discussion of this flu or influenza. The book takes a retrospective look at the flu with a view to infusing confidence in the modern people learning about the history of the plague. I hope by the time you're through with the book, you'll be able to learn from the past and deal more decisively with the future.

Chapter 1: The Brief History of the Spanish Flu

The year 1918 will never be forgotten in human history. Apart from being the year The Great War (later known as World War 1) ended, it was the year the deadly flu known as the Spanish flu broke out. It was a completely different flu that ravaged the world and defied all medical knowledge.

March 1918 to the spring of 1919 was a moment of panic, anxiety, and mourning. Viruses were known to kill. They were also known to be attacking the elderly and those with an underlying medical condition. But the Spanish flu had a completely different mode of operation. It seemed to target the seemingly healthy and agile young people between 25 to 40 years. This is not to say though that people outside that age bracket were completely spared.

What Is the Spanish Flu?

But what is the Spanish flu? Spanish flu or influenza is a highly contagious infectious disease caused by a flu virus. The deadly virus attacked the human respiratory system. It was transmitted through the droplets from the infected person when coughing, sneezing, or even talking. Because this virus is also airborne, anyone nearby an infected person can be infected by inhaling the virus.

Besides such direct human-to-human transmission, when a healthy person touches a surface or an object contaminated by the virus, the person is already carrying the virus on his or her hand. As soon that he or she touches his or her eyes, mouth, or with the hand, there was a great chance of becoming infected. No wonder the influenza was highly contagious.

The emergence of the Flu

No one could say for certainty when Spanish flu started. What we know is that it broke out simultaneously in many places. From the earliest reported cases, it is clear that the flu started sometime in March 1918.

Opinions also differ as to where the flu first struck. Some researchers point to China as the origin of the Spanish flu. But the more common position is that it began in Kansas in the Midwestern United States. Consider the first acceptable recorded cases which can be a pointer to its origin.

A pivotal date in the history of the Spanish flu was March 11, 1918, and it was in Fort Riley, a military outpost in Kansas. As usual, recruits were being hurriedly trained and oriented before going to battle in Europe. One of the cooks of the company, Albert Gitchel, came down with a sickness that was difficult to diagnose. The infirmary decided to put Gitchell on isolation for the bad flu, but not before others had been infected. This was taken to be the index case.

Less than an hour after isolating Gitchell, several soldiers began manifesting the same symptoms. All attempts to isolate these earliest carriers of the virus didn't prevent the flu from spreading. Almost everyone in Fort Riley was infected in quick succession. Within just five weeks, 1,127 have come down with what was later identified to be the Spanish flu and 46 of them finally died.

From there the flu found its way throughout the US, Europe. By May 1918, the French soldiers were seriously incapacitated by this flu. It later found its way to Russia, China, India, and far away, Africa, toward the end of July. By this time, people in all parts of the world were panicking because of what they didn't realize was the first wave of this influenza.

Why Called Spanish

You are unlikely to find a Spaniard feeling prejudiced against because deadly flu was erroneously given a name characterizing his nation. Though this might cause people erroneously conclude that the Spanish flu originated from Spain, historical facts prove otherwise.

It happened that Spain wasn't among the nations involved in the First World War. Allied countries and the Central Powers involved in the war campaign made deliberate efforts to underreport the damages of the war and were also covering up news of the flu to avoid dampening morale. But as a neutral country, the media in Spain was free to report on anything.

Thus, when the flu rampaged through the country, the Spanish government wasted no time in publicly declaring the presence of an epidemic. Since there was no censoring of Spanish health reports, many of the things that are initially known about the flu came through the Spanish media in Madrid. The flu thus came to be identified with the Spanish even though the Spaniards were reporting it as "French flu" with the belief that the virus came from France.

But there is another reason. The name "Spanish flu" was first used by the *British Medical Journal* to emphasize the effect of the disease on the Spaniards. It hit so hard in Spain to the extent that Spain's King Alfonso XIII was not spared. An in response, the Spaniards nicknamed the flu the "Naples Soldier". To German armies, it was *"Blitzkatarrh"* while the British troops described it as "Flanders grippe" and the "Spanish lady".

Spanish Flu Symptoms

The Spanish flu came in three waves. The world saw the first wave of the pandemic in the spring of 1918. It was generally mild with typical symptoms associated with common flu such as chills, fatigue, and fever with recovery taking place within a week. So the fatality rate was generally low.

The second wave was the real foe that surfaced about the fall of the same year. It was quite contagious and seemingly vengeful of the response to the first wave. It results in deaths within hours of striking its victims. More rugged victims endured only for days following the development of the earliest symptoms.

It was common for the skin of the victims to turn blue such that it would be difficult to determine the former color of their skin. Fluids were also found in their lungs that caused them to suffocate. The coughs induced by the flu were so persistent, forceful, and violent that the abdominal muscles of the victims tore. Foamy blood was flowing out of mouths and noses, and sometimes ears. Other symptoms were vomiting and incontinence. The third wave of the flu was less deadly.

But where did the flu come from? What caused it? And how many people were killed by the flu? The next chapter will answer the question.

Chapter 2: The Deadliest Plague in History

One hundred years after the flu, scientists could not say for certain where the flu originated from. Even though the first reported case was in the US, there are still theories pointing to France, China, or Britain as its origin.

Contrasting Figures, Piles of Dead

The origin is not the only thing unknown about the flu. The cause also was not known. H1N1 flu viruses were not new in 1918. They have been known to be attacking the very young and very old; making many of them sick and killing a number of them. Yes, other flu also killed in similar ways. But the Spanish flu mutated in 1918 into something more virulent and deadly.

While all agreed that it's the deadliest pandemic in history, the exact figure of the dead remains a subject of controversy. It was estimated to have infected about 500 million people worldwide while the world population was about 2 billion. At any rate, no one has given a figure below 20 million and above 100 million as the death toll.

It reportedly killed 25 million people in the first 25 weeks of its second wave. It was at this point the medical personnel who have been downplaying the flu as a small epidemic had to admit that it has spiraled out of control.

When international ports started letting in the infected to their countries, the infection had a free ride. A peculiarly serious case was reported in Sierra Leone where 500 out of 600 dock workers could not work because they all had caught the flu.

The truth is that the exact death toll is not known. Though the whopping number of 3 to 5 percent of the world population perished, there were no accurate medical records in many infected places, especially in African and Asian lands. In Tahiti, 10 percent of the entire population died in three weeks. 20 percent of Western Samoa suffered the same fate.

It went as far as wiping out families, decimating whole communities. Funeral parlors across the world were overwhelmed as there were piles of dead bodies to handle. And hospital personnel were helpless.

Remarkable Suddenness Worldwide

Commenting more recently on the suddenness with which the flu struck, the book author John M. Barry quotes an existing record of the event, saying: "In Rio de Janeiro, a man asked medical student Ciro Viera Da Cunha, who was waiting for a streetcar, for information in a perfectly normal voice, then fell down, dead; in Cape Town, South Africa, Charles Lewis boarded a streetcar for a three-mile trip home when the conductor collapsed, dead. In the next three miles six people aboard the streetcar died, including the driver."

What killed all of them? Even though all these died in different circumstances, they were killed by the same thing—the flu. And the deaths were sudden.

A Dearth of Vaccines and Medical Experts

Since the flu was so sudden with an unknown cause, it was difficult to find vaccines that could treat or even control it. Doctors and scientists weren't unsure of how to produce, recommend, or even administer antiviral. A number of them died while diagnosing or treating the victims due to the highly contagious nature of the disease.

Compounding the woes of the flu was the effect of World War 1 on the medical profession. Most of the countries involved in the war were left with a handful of physicians and health workers after many of them have perished in the war. There were not enough scientists to make research to unravel the cause and produce effective vaccines.

Downplaying the Seriousness

Some historians believe that the flu wouldn't have had such a fatality figure if politicians and medical personnel have taken it seriously. Rather than taking it for its potentials, they were underreporting it so as not to slow down the war efforts and keep boosting the troops' morale.

For instance, the *British Medical Journal* saw nothing wrong in overcrowding on transport and in the workplace even though this would contribute to the spread of the disease. It claimed that the then-ongoing war required that to be sustained and that the 'little inconvenience' created by the flu needed to be borne with 'dignity or patriotism'.

Individual doctors who should have spoken up were either unaware of the severity fully or were trying to curb the spread of anxiety and panic. Consider what happened in Cumbria, a former

Celtic kingdom in England. When the community medical officer saw the skyrocketing death rate, he requested that the rector stop ringing the church bells during funerals to reduce the awareness of another death and "keep people cheerful".

Probably due to the general censorship, the major press followed suit. *The Times* that was widely trusted in those days tried to make people look in the direction of "the general weakness of nerve-power known as war-weariness" instead of highlighting at the real picture. *The Manchester Guardian* taunted the calls for protective measures in these sarcastic words: "Women are not going to wear ugly masks."

Less Affected Areas and People

Despite all of these, there are a few areas that seemed immune to the flu. There were no reports of influenza deaths from those areas. However, could it also be that there were no accurate records?

An example of this is China that reportedly experienced relatively mild flu in 1918. However, experts believe that the report was due to a lack of a centralized collection of health statistics in China at the time. They claimed that some reports from the interior showed mortality rates from influenza that were perhaps higher in some locations in China.

Japan's case also was remarkable in the Spanish flu diary. It gave an estimated 0.4% mortality rate. Compared with almost all other Asian countries, this was very low. Again, it was attributed to inaccurate data. However, commendable was the effort of the Japanese government that severely restricted sea travel both domestic and international when the pandemic struck.

American Samoa and in the Pacific and the French colony of New Caledonia recorded a lesser fatality figure. While almost 12,000 Australian reportedly perished, these two lands effectively prevented even a single death from influenza. Their quarantines and isolation were prompt and effective.

Due to its isolated nature, the island of Marajó in Brazil's Amazon River Delta did not report an outbreak of flu by the end of the pandemic. There was no death reported also in St. Helena.

Even in lands that were seriously affected, children seemed to be protected in a special way. While adults and middle-aged people were fainting out of fear of an imminent flu attack in

19

1918, kids were seen skipping about without protective gear. Below was a typical song they were dancing to with their skipping ropes:

I had a little bird,

Its name was Enza.

I opened the window,

And in-flu-enza.

The story of the deadliness of the Spanish flu can conclude with this note from the *Journal of the American Medical Association,* December 28, 1918 (the final edition of the year)

"1918 has gone: a year momentous as the termination of the most cruel war in the annals of the human race; a year which marked, the end at least for a time, of man's destruction of man; unfortunately a year in which developed a most fatal infectious disease causing the death of hundreds of thousands of human beings. Medical science for four and one-half years devoted itself to putting men on the firing line and keeping them there. Now it must turn with its whole might to combating the greatest enemy of all--infectious disease."

What efforts were made to contain the disease? What were the aftermaths? What lessons can be learned from it? Can such lessons help to prevent an outbreak in the future? Please read on.

Chapter 3: The Spanish Flu and the Years After

The dawn of the 20th century was full of hope and aspirations. When you look at pictures of the era, it may strike us as quaint or even appealing. You could remember, for example, the time of horse-drawn carriages in the Western world. Top hats and long trailing skirts were in vogue.

Hardly would those pictures have anything in common with a terrifying worldwide march of death. The cause? Historians will tell you that the most destructive scourge in all recorded human history—the Spanish flu—destroyed not just humans during the 1918/1919 raid. It took a while before the world got near a recovery stage economically.

But first, let's take a look at efforts to contain the flu.

An Unforgettable Failure of Medical Scientists

Before the outbreak of the flu, medical science was making giant strides in putting diseases in check. In fact, during the war, doctors were receiving accolades and prided themselves in their ability to control and ultimately conquer any infectious disease. During the war, the journal *The Ladies Home* boasted that Americans no longer needed room to lay out their dead for view. It added the recommendation that such parlors henceforth renamed living rooms.

But the journal had to eat back its words when the Spanish flu struck. Historian Alfred W. Crosby writes: "All the physicians of 1918 were participants in the greatest failure of medical science in the twentieth century or, if absolute numbers of dead are the measure, of all time." Medical science failed woefully and had to swallow its pride. The lackadaisical attitudes of the politicians didn't help the matter as they sacrificed caution on the altar of the war campaign.

Fighting the Flu

Thanks to human resilience, people of those days didn't just fold their arms, lay low, and wait to be wiped away by as if by a global flood. They started taking precautions according to what they understood.

Since they knew it was transmittable through droplets and air from the infected, wearing of gloves and nose masks became the order of the day. Due to the alarming severity of the Spanish flu, people around the world were worried about getting it. In some cities, it was a crime to be found in the streets without wearing masks.

It was also an offense to spit, cough, or sneeze in public. *The New York Times* reported that Boy Scouts during the pandemic approached people spitting on the street in New York City and handed them cards reading: "You are in violation of the Sanitary Code."

Schools, theaters, and markets were close and all forms of public gatherings were prohibited. There were a lot of trials and errors in homemade prevention remedies. Eating of raw onions, keeping a potato in the pocket, or wearing a bag of camphor around the neck were all recommended as homemade remedies or preventions. But the deadly second wave of the influenza was too tough for any and all of these.

But the world was still not about to surrender.

Aspirin Came Promising but Poisoning

Instead of giving up since the flu defied all attempts to tame it, doctors began targeting its symptoms. Even if there was no cure in sight, they reasoned, the victims could have the symptoms alleviated. Thus, aspirin was called upon to come to the rescue.

The medication trademarked by Bayer in 1899 till 1917 got a new lease of life when other pharmaceutical companies started producing to meet the growing demand for it during the Spanish flu pandemic. The usage was adopted everywhere to treat and prevent influenza.

The U.S. Surgeon General, the U.S. Navy, and the *Journal of the American Medical Association* were among the respected authorities recommending the use of aspirin even before the spike in deaths allegedly caused by influenza. Unfortunately, aspirin couldn't live up to the expectation of the masses.

If anything, it hastened the death from the flu or caused fresh deaths. How so? Patients were advised by medical professionals to take as much as 30 grams per day! You know that was toxic if you put that side by side with current understanding that any dose above 4 grams of aspirin daily is unsafe. Using that much resulted in what was known as aspirin poisoning accompanying by hyperventilation and pulmonary edema. In fact, the buildup of fluid in the lungs was believed to be caused by aspirin poisoning.

Still, all hope was not lost.

Spanish Flu Pandemic Ends

Even though there was no known cure, the Spanish flu ended in 1919 summer. How? Efforts to reduce the spread paid off. Then bodies of those already infected later developed immunity while other victims died.

Since then, attempts have been made to explain what made the influenza virus so virulent. One of such was the discovery of a group of three genes that empowered the virus to overcome its victims' bronchial tubes and lungs. Bacterial pneumonia would then have a clear way to finish the havoc. The knowledge of this boosted the researcher's efforts to curb the flu.

The subsequent flu pandemics were not as deadly as the Spanish flu of 1918/1919 thanks to the lesson learned from behaviors and modes of transmission of viruses. These lessons will be the subject of the next chapter.

Chapter 4: Lessons From the Spanish Flu Outbreak

In 1997, at the small Eskimo village of Brevig, Alaska on the tundra of the Seward Peninsula, a scientist was examining the exhumed body of a young woman dug out of the permafrost by the four Eskimo helpers. The body was among the millions that fell to influenza back in then 1918, lain there, frozen, ever since.

Could the scientist learn anything from examining the body? Can we learn from whatever the scientist discovered? The scientist believed that the flu-causing agent could still be in her lungs. He hoped to employ advanced genetic engineering to isolate and identify the agent. The understanding of how viruses work lends credence to the viability of that project.

Some of the Lessons for Our Day

1. Give a pandemic the right name

Should the influenza of 1918 be named "Spanish flu" just because Spain exposed it and was hard hit by it? Well, Spain broke the conspiracy of silence which usually gives an opportunity to spread for pandemics. It has now become a common practice to misidentify illnesses as being from or belonging to a country, or an ethnic group.

This can weaken the efforts to garner worldwide supports for such pandemics as it was the case with the 2009 swine flu outbreak which was initially named "Mexican flu". The attention will be shifted to dealing with stigmatization and racism rather than the pandemic.

2. Let the public know the truth

The death toll from the Spanish flu might not be as high if authorities had concentrated on it and told the public the truth. They were concerned with keeping morale during the First World War when it hit. So, not wanting to allow any social disruptions that will negatively affect the war campaign, the authorities were giving untenable assurances that the flu was nothing more than a common cold.

When comparing that with the most recent pandemic, Mark Honigsbaum, a medical historian at City, University of London, said: "Epidemics all follow this similar arc where people deny or dismiss the threat until it becomes impossible to ignore any more." Giving knocks to the politicians giving false assurances, he added, "You still have politicians like Boris Johnson saying they're happy to shake hands. Just stop shaking hands. . . . We need to take this a little bit more seriously. I'm shocked by the complacency at the political level."

3. Control movements in times of epidemic

There were unusual movements during the pandemic of the First World War and this contributed to the severity of the scourge. Normally in a pandemic, the infected should be isolated and those suspected should be quarantined while the sickest should be in bed. But during the war, soldiers, included the infected but asymptomatic, were packed in trucks and were infecting one another. The infected and sick soldiers were simply sent home as nations struggle to strike a balance between their war interests and public health. These continued to infect others as many as they came in contact with and the disease continued to spread.

Governments should not hesitate to impose lockdown and temporarily clampdown on civil life to reduce human to human infection of diseases. Public health should be placed above all sentimental considerations.

4. All should beware of a second wave

If the countries didn't let down their guards after the first wave of Spanish flu, it wouldn't have been that bad because the death rate was initially small. However, governments and health workers were not on the watch when the second wave broke out by August 1918. The virus had mutated and came to become a far deadlier form. It hit hardest in parts of the world that had not already been exposed by the first wave and low immunity.

Thus, while rejoicing in containing any flu virus infection, efforts should be made to prevent its resurgence. Thus, flu vaccines should be given annually.

Another Pandemic Coming?

A research work by London's National Institute for Medical Research states: "In some ways, conditions prevail as they did in 1918: there is a huge volume of international travel due to the development of transport, there are a number of war-zones with their inherent problems of malnutrition and poor hygiene, the world population has grown to six and a half billion and a greater proportion of this population is living in urban situations many of which have decaying infrastructures in terms of waste disposal."

Commenting on the possibility flu, an article in the medical journal *Vaccine* submitted in 2003: "It has been 35 years since the last influenza pandemic, and the longest interval between pandemics recorded with certainty is 39 years . . . . The pandemic virus may emerge in China or a nearby country and could include surface antigens or virulence factors derived from animal influenza viruses."

Summing all of these up you can agree with experts that it's not a matter of if virus flu will return, but it's about when and how it will.

Predicting concerning the next flu virus, *Vaccine* continued: "It will spread rapidly throughout the world. Several waves of infection will occur. Morbidity will be extensive in all age groups, and there will be widespread disruption of social and economic activity in all countries. Excess mortality will be evident in most if not all age groups. It is unlikely that health care systems in even the most economically developed countries will be able to adequately cope with the demand for health care services."

Avoiding the Next Pandemic

The best defense against the next flu is to take to heart the lessons learned from the previous flu infections. The next thing is to anticipate an outbreak before it occurs. The above facts show that the next pandemic is just around the corner. The consciousness of this should move medical experts to intensify their research and governments to stockpile vaccines and whatever is needed to nip infections at the bud.

It's the collective responsibilities of the government and individuals. Living in squalors with limited access to vaccines, clean water, sanitation, and healthcare facilities is a disaster in the making. Efforts should be made to avoid this. Poverty is a vehicle of transmission of diseases. Government and private sectors should concentrate on poverty eradication.

Hygiene and a good diet should continue to be preached. All and sundry should work toward boosting their body's immune system to improve its response to infections.

Then the world will be ready to prevent or curb the next epidemic.

CONCLUSIONS

You may not have met those widowed by the Spanish flu of 1918. But there are chances you would meet or hear a more recent comment directly from those orphaned by it. You will then see that all that has been written about the full is not capable of describing what actually happened.

This book presents a nice summary and a vivid picture of what happened within those gruesome months. It is hoped that the lessons you've learned here will give an added proof to all stakeholders in disease management including but not limited to you.

Manufactured by Amazon.ca
Bolton, ON